Autoimmune Protocol Made Simple Cookbook

50 Gluten Free, Paleo Recipes For Healthy Living

Compiled by

Lourie Harrold

Copyright ©2020

All rights reserved

This book is for public consumption, any reproduction of any parts of this book must be done with written permission from the publisher.

DISCLAIMER

Information contained in this book is not written with the intent to recommend any medical or nutritional advice. Any nutritional course of action you take on should be discussed with your doctor first. The information in this book is based solely on personal experiences and research.

ACKNOWLEDGMENT

Special thanks to the wonderful people that i got some of the pictorial illustrations in this book.

Dedication

To everybody managing an autoimmune condition. Stay strong.

Contents

- INTRODUCTION 10
- CHAPTER 1 12
  - For Starters: What is this Autoimmune Topic All About 12
    - What is an Autoimmune Disease? 12
    - A List of Some of the Most Common Autoimmune Diseases 13
    - Tests/Diagnosis for Autoimmune Diseases 15
  - The Paleo Autoimmune Protocol (AIP) Diet 17
- CHAPTER 2 19
  - Breakfast Recipes 19
    - 1. Chicken and Apple Sausages 20
    - 2. Carrot and Apple Hash with Cinnamon and Ginger 22
    - 3. Thyme Breakfast Cookies 23
    - 4. Sweet Potato Porridge with Fresh Berries 24
    - 5. Coconut Banana Pancakes Topped with Berries and Coconut Cream 25
    - 6. Bacon Zucchini Mushroom Spinach No-Egg Scramble 26
    - 7. Kale Green Smoothie with Avocado and Banana 27
- CHAPTER 2 28
  - Salad Recipes 28
    - 1. Citrus Avocado Salad 29
    - 2. Mango and Chicken Salad with Coconut Caesar Dressing 31
    - 3. Strawberry Salad with Shredded Carrot 32
    - 4. Simple Garlic Cucumber Salad 33
    - 5. Steak Kale Salad with Coconut Pan-Fried Peaches 34
- CHAPTER 3 35
  - Soup Recipes 35
    - 1. Salmon Stew with Celery and Cilantro 37
    - 2. Simple Slow Cooker Bone Broth 38

    3. Slow Cooker Thai Chicken Soup 39

    4. Coconut Seafood Soup 40

    5. Spaghetti Squash Soup with Apple 41

CHAPTER 3 43

Entree Recipes 43

    1. Slow Cooker Pal Beef Stew 44

    2. Slow Cooker Bacon and Chicken 45

    3. Pineapple Pork with Garlic and Cilantro 46

    4. Pan-Fried Tilapia with Coconut Carrot Mash and Garlic Zucchini Sauté 47

    5. Pan-Fried Pork Tenderloin with Peach and Basil Sauce 48

    5. Grilled Chicken Drumsticks with Garlic Marinade 49

    6. Saffron Orange Acorn Squash Mash with Bacon and Collard Greens 50

    7. Braised Cardamom Cabbage and Pork 51

    8. Thai Chicken and Cauliflower Rice 52

    9. Cauliflower Crusted Pizza topped with Spinach and Prosciutto 53

    10. Baked Salmon on a bed of Cabbage, Fennel, and Apple 55

CHAPTER 4 56

Side Dish Recipes 56

    1. Ginger and Garlic Bok Choy Sauté 57

    2. Endives and Pear Sauté 58

    3. Roasted Turmeric Cauliflower 59

    4. Easy Bacon Brussels Sprouts 60

    5. Lemon Asparagus Sauté with Bacon Topping 61

    6. Baked Parsnip Fries with Parsley 62

    7. Coconut Mashed Sweet Potatoes with Shredded Coconut and Ginger 63

CHAPTER 5 64

Snack Recipes 64

    1. Baked Sweet Potato Chips 65

    2. Avocado Bacon Cups 66

    3. Dehydrated Fruits and Vegetables 68

    4. Coconut Plantains Chips 69

    5. Salt and Vinegar Kale Chips 70

CHAPTER 6 71
Dessert 71
- 1. Raw Carrot Cake 72
- 2. Apple Ginger Spice Sweet Potato Cookies 73
- 3. Cinnamon Pear and Butternut Squash Bowls 74
- 4. 5-Minute Pumpkin Pie 75
- 5. Microwave Banana Bread 76
- 6. Strawberry Banana Macaroons 77
- 7. Vanilla Coconut Blueberry Bars 78
- 8. Berry Jello 79
- 9. Coconut Butter Stuffed Dates 80
- 10. Pineapple Mango Banana Sorbet 81

FOREWARD

My name is Laurie Hendon, and i compiled this to help fellow comrades in the fight of managing their autoimmune conditions and healing their bodies through healthy living.

You are not alone in the fight.

INTRODUCTION

Having The Right Food To Eat Is The Way To Good Health

I've adored eating for as long as i can recollect. In any case, for the greater part of my life, I cherished eating junk, or if nothing else processed food items. All things considered, there's no denying that most junk food is truly addictive. Yet, in my battles to recuperate my body after finding out i had an Autoimmune disease, including my digestion, it was my chance to Paleo and Real Food that had more effect than everything else.

When I at long last comprehended the effect food had on my body, I immediately figured out how to acknowledge and cherish genuine, whole, fresh food sources. What's more, today, I sense that I eat like better ever seen, both as far as health and taste. What's more, similarly as critically, I typically anticipate cooking, which was never the situation when I was more youthful. Indeed, even 5 years back, I saw cooking as a task that would occupy what little time I had, instead of an enjoyment and energizing chance to make delectable food and cause myself to feel better.

Furthermore, that is the thing that I need to have the option to impart to you and share with the world.

A Love for Cooking, with a Little Perspective

I despised cooking for most of my life. And for years, I worked long hours as a banker in New York City, so I had exceptionally small interest or time to cook after getting home from a long day at the office. In other words, I get it totally that cooking may not be the primary thing you see forward to each morning, midday, and evening. But however, I know that everyone can learn to appreciate it. I accept it's an action that can bring companions and family together like few others. And I believe that it doesn't got to be amazingly complicated or time-consuming. Most of all, if you've got an autoimmune disease, I believe that cooking is one of the foremost vital and effective things you can do to recuperate your body and begin living a life you love. And that's why I composed this cookbook for a Paleo Autoimmune Diet.

Getting your Body to Heal Can Be Fun and Easy

It probably won't be exact to state that healing your body is simple each and every day, except it shouldn't be a long lasting battle. Also, everything begins in the kitchen. Indeed there are some stunning eateries and some extraordinary food points out there however 99% of cafés and processed food are suspects of unhealthy eating to mildly put it. In the event that you're attempting to heal an autoimmune disease, at that point practically the entirety of the daily diet you eat should be cooked at home. But honestly, that is hard if every meal is taking hours to get ready or on the off chance that you can't buy the ingredients at your local grocery store.

I think Recipes shouldn't be hard but Simple and Easy

It sounds senseless, yet I figure most recipes ought to be basic, quick, and simple. On extraordinary events, I once in a while decide to make complex and tedious dishes. Be that as it may, on ordinary days, I don't have the enough time or strength to fix up an elaborate meal after the day's work. With only a few special cases, the entirety of the recipes I'm going to show you now are exceptionally simple to make, they don't take a lot of time, and they turn out well every single time. In such a case that any of these things isn't valid, at that point cooking rapidly turns out to be more of a stress. What's more, on the off chance that cooking turns out to be less fun, at that point we're substantially more likeable to return to eating food that don't heal or sustain our bodies. And i know absolutely that, that's not what anybody managing an autoimmune disease would want.

How about we Build a Better Life

This is only a cookbook. In any case, I see it as considerably more than that. I see this as an open door for you to significantly improve your wellbeing and your life. An opportunity to assume responsibility for your body and feel more youthful, more beneficial, and more joyful. A large portion of all, I see it as an instrument for you to carry on with an actual existence that you love.

CHAPTER 1

For Starters: What is this Autoimmune Topic All About

What is an Autoimmune Disease?

The first time someone told me they had an autoimmune disease, I was quite clueless and thought they meant something chronically life threatening and i felt terribly emotional about it. Obviously, I was wrong.

An autoimmune disease is a condition whereby your body's immune system attacks other parts of your body (instead of attacking foreign invaders like germs). The effects are varied, but these diseases often result in widespread destruction of organs and cells. The immune system normally guards against germs and foreign bodies like bacteria and viruses. When it senses these foreign bodies, it dispatches a troop of soldier cells to attack them and defend the body. On an average, the immune system of the body can always differentiate between alien cells and your own cells.

However, in an autoimmune disease, the immune system tends to mistake part of it's own healthy own body, like the bones or maybe skin, as foreign and harmful. It then sends out substances called autoantibodies that attack healthy cells. Although it can be seen that some autoimmune diseases target only one organ, there are still others that attack the whole body. For example, Type 1 diabetes damages the pancreas. Other diseases, like systemic lupus erythematosus (SLE), commonly called Lupus affect the whole body.

How is it possible that the immune system can attack it's own body?

Doctors and scientists are yet to find out exactly what causes the immune-system attacking it's own body. Yet some group or classes people are more liable to develop an autoimmune disease than others. Let's look at these groups categorically.

1. **Gender**: A survey was carried out in 2014, and it was discovered that women get autoimmune diseases more than men at a rate of about 2 to 1 compared to men — 6.4 percent of women against 2.7 percent of that of men. Often the disease starts during a woman's childbearing year ie between 15-45 of age..

2. **Race/Ethnicity**: Some autoimmune diseases are more common and tend to occur more often in certain ethnic groups. For example, lupus is more popular in African-American and Hispanic people than Caucasians.
3. **Weight**: Excess weight or obesity increases risk of having rheumatoid arthritis or psoriatic arthritis. A reason could be that having more weight puts greater stress on the joints or because fat tissue makes substances that increases the chances joint capsule inflammation.
4. **Smokers**: Research carried out among smoking Autoimmune Diseases patients has linked smoking to a number of autoimmune diseases, including lupus, rheumatoid arthritis, hyperthyroidism and MS.
5. **Also**, certain medications especially blood pressure medications or antibiotics can trigger drug-induced lupus, which is often a more benign form of lupus. Some medications used to lower cholesterol, called statins, can trigger statin-induced myopathy (weakness of the muscle). Before one starts or stops any medications, it's pertinent to make a visit to the hospital and try to talk to your doctor.
6. **Certain autoimmune diseases**, like multiple sclerosis and lupus, are hereditary and run in families. It will necessarily mean that all members of the family will have the same disease, but they inherit a susceptibility to an autoimmune disease. Because the cases of autoimmune diseases is on rise each every year, researchers suspect environmental factors like infections and exposure to chemicals or solvents might also be involved.
7. **A "diet of highly processed food"** is another suspected risk factor for developing an autoimmune disease. Due to the fast paced nature of the modern world, most people are condemned to this averse diet.Eating mostly high-fat, high-sugar, and highly processed foods is thought to be linked to inflammation, which might set off an immune response. However, this theory hasn't been proven by scientists.

In 2015, a survey was carried out with the hypothesis on another theory called the hygiene hypothesis. For the reason of vaccination and antiseptics, most children born today aren't exposed to as many germs as children born earlier in the years were in the past. The lack of exposing maybe had made their immune system prone to acting against harmless substances.

A List of Some of the Most Common Autoimmune Diseases

- Hashimoto's Thyroiditis
- Graves' disease
- Type 1 Diabetes
- Rheumatoid Arthritis

- Psoriasis
- Celiac Disease
- Crohn's Disease
- Lupus
- Narcolepsy
- Ulcerative Colitis
- Multiple Sclerosis
- Guillain-Barré Syndrome
- HidradenitisSuppurativa
- Alopecia Areata
- Autoimmune Hepatitis
- Angioedema

General Symptoms of Autoimmune diseases

The early symptoms of many autoimmune diseases are more often than not similar bin nature, they may include the following:

- Numbness and tingling in the hands and feet
- Hair loss
- Skin rashes
- Swelling and redness
- Low-grade fever
- Trouble concentrating
- Fatigue
- Achy muscles

Some of the diseases can also have their own distinct symptoms, and symptoms may also vary in different persons. For example, type 1 diabetes causes extreme thirst, weight loss, and fatigue. IBD causes belly pain, bloating, and diarrhea.

With autoimmune diseases like Psoriasis or RA, symptoms may come and go. A period of symptoms is called a flare-up. A time when the symptoms go away is called remission.

With autoimmune diseases like psoriasis or RA, symptoms may come and go. A period of symptoms is called a flare-up. A period when the symptoms go away is called remission.

When is it time to visit the hospital

Make sure to see a doctor if you have symptoms of an autoimmune disease. You might need to visit a specialist, depending on the type of disease you have.

Rheumatologists are specialist doctors that treat joint diseases, like rheumatoid arthritis as well as other autoimmune diseases like Sjögren's syndrome and SLE.

Gastroenterologists are specialist doctors that treat conditions of the GI tract, such as celiac and Crohn's disease.

Endocrinologists are specialist doctors treat diseases of the glands, including Graves' disease, Hashimoto's thyroiditis, and Addison's disease.

Dermatologists treat skin infections and diseases and , such as psoriasis.

Tests/Diagnosis for Autoimmune Diseases

No single examination can clearly diagnose most autoimmune diseases. Your doctor will use a combination of tests and a review of your symptoms, family history and physical examination to diagnose you. A very popular test is the ANA. The antinuclear antibody test (ANA) is often one of the first tests that doctors use when symptoms suggest an autoimmune disease. A positive test means you may have one of these diseases, but it wont be able to clearly state exactly which oneof the disease you have or if you have one for sure. Other tests look for specific autoantibodies produced in certain autoimmune diseases. Your doctor might also do nonspecific tests to check for the inflammation these diseases produce in the body.

Treatment: How are autoimmune diseases treated?

Treatments can't cure autoimmune conditions, but they can suppress to an extent, the overactive immune response and bring down inflammation or at least reduce pain and inflammation. Drugs used to treat these conditions include: nonsteroidal anti-inflammatory drugs (NSAIDs), such as ibuprofen (Motrin, Advil) and naproxen (Naprosyn) immune-suppressing drugs. Treatments are also available to relieve symptoms like pain, swelling, fatigue, and skin rashes. Eating a well-balanced diet and getting regular exercise may also help you feel better. Autoimmune Diseases also increases your chances of developing other disease conditions. For example, having lupus, rheumatoid arthritis or psoriatic arthritis raises your risk for heart disease. While taking steps to reduce heart disease is always a good idea, it is even more essential if unfortunately you have any of these conditions. Discuss with your physician about what can done to keep your heart healthy and strong. For example, keeping your blood pressure and cholesterol levels within healthy ranges, eating a nutritious diet and exercising regularly can be lifesaving.

How does Food come into the picture?

Our intestines are lined with epithelial cells designed to keep most substances out of our bloodstream and to allow other substances in (like digested food). However, for a variety of reasons, those epithelial cells can become either damaged or confused, in which case they start letting too many things pass into our bloodstream.

Bacteria and dietary antigens can then pass into our bloodstream, causing our bodies' immune system to attack them. This is generally a good thing, since that's how we fight off illness and infection. However, if that happens often enough, then our immune system often starts attacking other parts of our body, rather than just the foreign invaders. And that's when an autoimmune disease is born. Food is incredibly important to this whole process, because it's one of the primary things that can cause the epithelial cells in our intestines to become or remain damaged and confused.

The Paleo Autoimmune Protocol (AIP) Diet

The (AIP) diet is a generally new, food based way to deal with dispensing with undesirable pain and inflammation in an individual's body. It's an eating routine that is thought to help help your gut to lessen aggravation made via by Autoimmune conditions. It's a variation of a Paleo diet to help those with autoimmune diseases. In particular, foods that can "irritate and damage the intestines of some people" must be eliminated for a time and then reintroduced to see how your particular body reacts. The eating routine is exceptionally prohibitive and predominantly incorporates meats and vegetables. For the most part, you would attempt the AIP diet for a little while before including food outside of the eating routine. If you have an autoimmune disease - and if a Paleo or Real Food diet has not completely cleared up your symptoms - then it's about time you go for a change by trying a Paleo Autoimmune Protocol. I must also add it requires a commitment. Trying it for just 4-5 days is NOT going to help. It takes time and discipline to properly heal. And because the protocol is more restrictive, it's best to ensure you don't eat out at all during that period.

Four Vital Steps To Healing

For you to check your development, these 4 steps are vital

1. Discpline yourself: this maybe cliche but it's just the plain truth, you need to fully admit that it's going to be a bit of a lifestyle change for the next few months and probably for the rest of your life. Tell your family, friends and colleagues what you're doing and why, so that they'll help and support you and not wonder why you would all of a sudden start dodging eating out with them or rejecting their food gift packs. It might appear rude to them.

2. 2 months of Elimination. This is where this cookbook comes in. For 2 months, you need to eliminate all foods that may be causing you problems.

3. Start Re-Introducing One Food at a Time. After 2 months, continue to cook meals with no potentially problematic ingredients. Start from the ones you feel very comfortable with. However, start introducing one ingredient for a few days at a time.

4. Make sure to keep notes and evaluate how you feel. Keep a list of foods that make you feel worse when you reintroduce them and a list of foods that don't make you feel worse. Then keep going through ingredients until you know exactly which foods cause you trouble. If you need to, repeat steps 1-4 every year or so, as the results will often change over time.

Common Mistakes on a Paleo Autoimmune Protocol

There are 2 common mistakes that people make on a Paleo Autoimmune Protocol:

1. Changing of Diet Only

Stress, lack of sleep, and lack of exercise (or too much exercise for some people) are huge components of AIP that many people miss. It's all whole lifestyle change, so you have to discuss with your doctor to streamline your daily activities to how best it can be for your health.

2. Eating Foods that You're Sensitive To.

Even if a certain food is permitted on AIP, you might still be sensitive to it (e.g., coconut products). So, if you know or suspect there's something else you should be avoiding, then just treat it as a "not allowed" food and reintroduce it after the elimination period.

Lastly, remember that although the 50 recipes in this book are designed to help you enjoy AIP and to make it as easy and painless as possible, they won't be replicas of what you used to eat. Clearly, pizza is not going to taste the same without tomato sauce, cheese, and a gluten-filled crust! But there are plenty of comfort foods in this book as well as recipes that will open your palate to new flavors and your mind to new ideas. Keep an open mind, be ready to experiment some, and most importantly, start enjoying some amazing real foods that will heal your body.

CHAPTER 2

Breakfast Recipes

This section includes seven easy and simple recipes that will make your morning great.

Let's go!

1. Chicken and Apple Sausages

Estimated time for preparation: 30 minutes

Output: Twelve pieces of sausages

Servings: Four Servings

Ingredients:

- 1 tablespoon fresh thyme leaves, finely cut or use 2 tablespoons dried thyme
- 3 tablespoons fresh parsley, finely chopped
- 1 tablespoon fresh oregano, finely chopped (or use 2 tablespoons dried oregano)
- 2 large chicken breasts, or use 1 lb ground chicken meat
- 1 apple, peeled and finely diced
- 2 teaspoons garlic powder
- salt and pepper as you prefer
- coconut oil

Mode of Preparation:

1. Preheat oven to 425F.

2. Place 3 tablespoons of coconut oil into a skillet and cook (on a medium-high heat) the apples, thyme, parsley, and oregano until the apples soften (cook for about 7-8 minutes).

3. Remove the skillet from heat and let it cool for 5-7 minutes.

4. Food process the chicken breast (if you're not using ground chicken meat).

5. Put the chicken in a mixing bowl and combine the chicken meat with everything in the skillet as well as the garlic powder, salt and pepper including any leftover oil.

6. Form 12 thin patties (1/2 inch thick) from the meat and place on a baking tray lined with foil (so you don't need to wash the baking tray).

7. Bake the patties for about 20 minutes. Check with a meat thermometer that the internal temperature of a patty near the middle of the tray is 170F.

8. If you want the sausages to be browned, then just pan-fry for a few minutes in coconut oil.

9. Alternatively, if you don't want to bake, you can also pan-fry the raw sausages instead of putting them into the oven.

10. Cool and store in fridge or freezer. You can always eat out of it in some hours time or even the next morning, just reheat easily in the skillet or in the microwave.

11. Enjoy your morning!

2. Carrot and Apple Hash with Cinnamon and Ginger

Estimated time for preparation: 20 minutes

Output: Two plates

Servings: Two

Ingredients:

- Coconut oil for cooking
- cinnamon (for sprinkling)
- fresh ginger, for topping
- 1 medium carrot, grated or shredded
- 1 apple, peeled and grated or shredded

Mode of preparation:

1. Make sure to remove dripping water from the carrots and apples.

2. Turn the apples and carrots shred together and pour 3 tablespoons of coconut oil into the frying-pan.

3. Form 2 large flat patties in the frying-pan and fry on medium heat. Fry each side for about 2-3 minutes and be careful when turning. Make sure to check it doesn't burn.

4. Serve with a sprinkling of cinnamon and freshly grated ginger.

5. Enjoy your morning!

3. Thyme Breakfast Cookies

Estimated Time for preparation: 40 minutes

Output: Six-eight cookies

Servings: 2-3

Ingredients:

- 6 tablespoons olive oil
- 1/4 cup cooked bacon pieces
- 1/2 cup coconut flour
- 1/2 teaspoon baking powder
- 1 teaspoon thyme

Mode of Preparation:

1. Heat up your oven to 350F.

2. Mix all the ingredients together and divide to form 6-8 small cookies.

3. Spread each part on parchment paper.

4. Bake for about 20-25 minutes until golden

You can see that there are no eggs in this recipe, the absence of eggs makes the cookies crumbly, so take care to be steady when picking them up.

5. Enjoy your morning!

4. Sweet Potato Porridge with Fresh Berries

Estimated Time for Preparation: 20 minutes

Output: 3-4 cups

Servings: 4

Ingredients:

- 3 tablespoons coconut oil
- 2 medium cooked sweet potatoes (boil, bake, or microwave them or use 1 14oz can of sweet potato or butternut squash puree)
- Dash of cloves
- Handful of fresh berries
- 1 tablespoon shredded coconut
- 1 cup coconut milk
- 1 teaspoon cinnamon
- ½ teaspoon nutmeg

Directions:

1. Put the sweet potatoes in a blender and blend the sweet potatoes, coconut milk, coconut oil, cinnamon, nutmeg, and cloves together.

2. Pour into a small pot and heat the mixture midly.

3. Add the fresh berries and shredded coconut on top.

4. Enjoy you morning!

5. Coconut Banana Pancakes Topped with Berries and Coconut Cream

Estimated Time for Preparation: 20 minutes

Output: Seven pancakes

Servings: Two

Ingredients:

- Coconut oil for cooking
- Fresh berries
- Coconut cream (from the top of a can of refrigerated coconut milk)
- 2 ripe bananas
- 1/3 cup coconut flour
- 1 teaspoon vanilla extract
- 1/2 teaspoon baking powder

Directions:

1. Mix the coconut flour, vanilla extract, bananas, and baking powder and mix well.

2. Add in 3-4 tablespoons of coconut oil into a frying pan on low to medium heat.

3. Scoop out about 2-3 full tablespoons of batter for each pancake and spread the batter to form a thin pancake (1/4 to 1/2 inch thick).

4. Fry each side for 2-3 minutes until it's a bit solid and browns. It's pertinent to note that it burns easily so use a low heat.

5. Fry the pancakes. Depending on the size of your frying pan, you can fry all at once or you can fry them in batches.

6. Top with fresh berries and coconut cream.

7. Enjoy your morning!!

6. Bacon Zucchini Mushroom Spinach No-Egg Scramble

Estimated Time For Preparation: 20 minutes

Output: Two large bowls

Servings: 2

Ingredients:

- Handful of spinach, washed
- 10 slices of bacon (chopped)
- 1 tablespoon coconut oil
- 2 zucchinis, sliced (1/2 inch thick) and quartered
- 10 baby Portobello mushrooms, sliced (or use other mushrooms)

Directions:

1. On a chopping board, chop up the zucchinis, mushrooms, and the bacon and keep them separately in different plates.

2. Add 1 tablespoon of coconut oil to the frying pan.

3. Then Add the chopped zucchinis and mushrooms to the frying pan and cook on medium heat.

4. Fry the bacon pieces in a separate pot until perfectly done.

5. Add the cooked bacon pieces to the frying pan. Cook for 2 minutes more in the frying pan.

6. Add the spinach to the frying pan and for another 2 minutes.

7. Enjoy your morning!!

7. Kale Green Smoothie with Avocado and Banana

Estimated Time for Preparation: 5 minutes

Output: 2 glasses

Servings: 2

Ingredients:

- 1 1/2 cups coconut milk
- Handful of baby kale (or spinach)
- 2 tablespoons of coconut oil
- 1 avocado
- 2 bananas
- 1/2 cup frozen berries (or fresh berries)

Directions:

1. Blend well. Combine all ingredients in a blender and pulse until smooth.

2. Enjoy your morning!!

CHAPTER 2

Salad Recipes

This section includes five easy and simple recipes that are tasty and good for your health.

Let's go!

1. Citrus Avocado Salad

Estimated Time for Preparation: 10 minutes

Output: 1 small bowl

Servings: 2

Ingredients:

- 2 tablespoons of olive oil
- 1 tablespoon of balsamic vinegar
- Salt and pepper, to taste
- 2 ripe avocados, pitted and cubed
- 1/2 grapefruit, peeled and cubed
- 1/2 navel orange, peeled and cubed

Directions:

1. Mix and turn all the ingredients well.
2. Enjoy your salad

2. Mango and Chicken Salad with Coconut Caesar Dressing

Estimated Time for Preparation: 30 minutes

Output: 1 large salad bowl

Servings: 2

Ingredients:

- 1/2 cup coconut cream (cream from the top of a refrigerated can of coconut milk)
- 2 tablespoons coconut oil
- 2 cloves garlic (or garlic powder)
- 1 head of romaine lettuce, washed and chopped
- 2 chicken breasts, diced
- Coconut oil to cook with
- 1 mango, peeled and diced
- Salt and Pepper

Directions:

1. Blend the coconut cream, coconut oil, garlic, and salt and pepper to make a salad cream.

2. Add 2 tablespoons of coconut oil into a frying pan. Cook the diced chicken in the frying pan. Add salt and pepper to your taste.

3. Toss the romaine lettuce, chicken breast, and diced mango in the salad cream.

4. Enjoy your salad

3. Strawberry Salad with Shredded Carrot

Estimated Time for preparation: 10 minutes

Output: 1 large bowl

Servings: 4

Ingredients

- 3 strawberries
- 1/3 cup of olive oil
- 2 tablespoons of apple cider vinegar
- 2 oz (approx. 4-6 handfuls) baby spinach leaves, washed
- 10 medium sized strawberries, sliced
- 1/2 carrot, shredded

Instructions

1. In a blender, blend the 3 strawberries, olive oil, and apple cider vinegar to make the a fine pulp.

2. Toss pulp with the spinach, sliced strawberries, and shredded carrot.

3. Enjoy your salad!!

4. Simple Garlic Cucumber Salad

Estimated Time for preparation: 10 minutes

Output: 2-3 cups

Servings: 2

Ingredients

- 2 tablespoons olive oil
- Dill for sprinkling (optional)
- 1 large cucumber, peeled
- 6 cloves garlic, minced
- Salt to taste

Instructions

1. Cut the cucumber into cubes.
2. Toss the cucumbers with the minced garlic, salt, and olive oil.
3. Best served chilled. Sprinkle dill on top.
4. Enjoy your salad

5. Steak Kale Salad with Coconut Pan-Fried Peaches

Estimated Time for preparation: 30 minutes

Yield: Two plates

Servings: 2

Ingredients:

- 2 peaches (white or yellow), slice off 2 large slices and dice the rest
- 1 6-8oz filet mignon beef steaks (or other steaks), sliced in half to make 2 thinner steaks
- Coconut oil for cooking
- 3 handfuls of baby kale, washed
- Salt and pepper, to taste
- Olive oil and balsamic vinegar for dressing

Directions:

1. Grill or pan-fry (using coconut oil) the thin steaks and the peach pieces.

2. Toss the kale with the cooked diced peach and season with salt, pepper, olive oil, and balsamic vinegar to taste.

3. Put the steaks on top of the kale salad and dress with the bigger peach piece.

4. Enjoy your salad!!

CHAPTER 3

Soup Recipes

This chapter has 5 amazing recipes for you to enjoy.

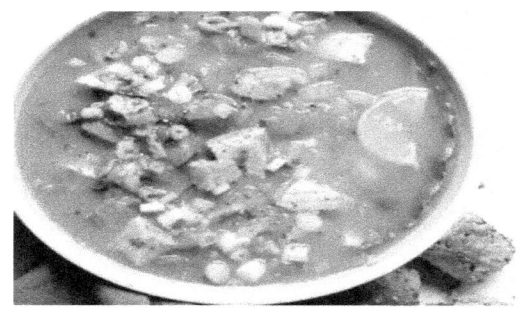

www.my24recipes.com

1. Salmon Stew with Celery and Cilantro

Estimated Time for preparation: 30 minutes

Yield: Four bowls

Servings: 4

Ingredients:

- 2 salmon filets, diced
- 2 Italian squash, diced
- 4 button mushrooms, diced
- 2 cups chopped celery
- 1/2 cup chopped cilantro
- 32oz chicken broth (or bone broth)
- salt and pepper (to taste)

Directions:

1. Put all the vegetables with the broth into a pot and heat for about 15 minutes.

2. Then add the diced salmon and simmer for another 5 minutes.

3. Soup is ready

2. Simple Slow Cooker Bone Broth

Estimated Time for preparation: 8 hours

Yield: Eleven bowls

Servings: 10

Ingredients:

- 1/2 cup parsley, chopped
- 3 garlic, minced
- 1 teaspoon grated ginger
- 2 ribs of celery, chopped
- 3-4 lbs of bones
- 1 gallon water (or as much as will fit into the slow cooker)
- 2 tablespoons apple cider vinegar

Directions:

1. Add all the ingredients to the crockpot.

2. Cook on low setting in crockpot for 8+ hours (longer is better).

3. Allow the broth to cool, strain and pour broth into container.

4. Store in refrigerator.

5. Scoop out the congealed fat on top of the broth if you want.

6. Heat broth when needed, add seasoning to taste.

3. Slow Cooker Thai Chicken Soup

Estimated Time for preparation: 8 hours

Yield: 10+ bowls

Servings: 10

Ingredients:

- 20 fresh basil leaves (10 for the slow cooker, and 10 for garnish)
- 5 thick slices of fresh ginger
- 1 lime
- 1 whole chicken
- 1 stalk of lemongrass, cut into large chunks
- 1 tablespoon salt
- Additional salt to taste

Directions:

1. Put the poultry, lemongrass, 10 basil leaves, ginger, and salt into the slow cooker. And fill up with water

2. Cook on low for 8-10 hours.

3. Ladle the broth into a bowl, add in salt to taste, squeeze in fresh lime juice to taste, and garnish with chopped basil leaves.

4. Enjoy!!

4. Coconut Seafood Soup

Estimated Time for preparation: 30 minutes

Output: Four big bowls

Servings: 4

Ingredients:

- 4 tilapia filets, chopped into large chunks
- 10 shrimp/prawns
- 10 mussels, optional
- 1 cup coconut cream
- 32oz chicken stock (or water)
- 10 mushrooms (or other mushrooms), sliced
- 1/2 cup kale, chopped
- 1 cup romaine lettuce, chopped
- 1 teaspoon Red Boat fish sauce
- Salt

Directions:

1. Add in the mushrooms, kale, and romaine lettuce, and heat till it boils.

2. Pour the chicken stock into a large pot and heat till it boils.

3. Add in the tilapia pieces, the shrimp/prawns, and any other seafood, and bring to the boil again. Ensure the soup covers all the seafood.

4. Heat for around 4 minutes until the seafood have turned pink and the tilapia pieces are no longer translucent.

5. Add in the coconut cream, fish sauce (if you like), and salt to taste. Stir carefully to mix.

6. Wait for it to just start boiling, then take off the heat and serve immediately.

7. Enjoy your soup!

5. Spaghetti Squash Soup with Apple

Estimated Time for preparation: 40 minutes

Output: 4 bowls

Servings: 4

Ingredients:

- 16oz chicken stock (or water)
- 2 teaspoons cinnamon
- 1 spaghetti squash
- 1 apple, cored and peeled and cut into chunks
- dash of nutmeg
- dash of cloves
- salt to taste

Directions:

1. Remove the outer skin and the seeds of the spaghetti squash.

2. Cut the spaghetti squash into chunks.

3. Pour the chicken stock into a large pot and heat to boil

4. Place the apple chunks and the spaghetti squash chunks into the pot, and cook until the squash is very tender.

5. Use an immersion blender to puree the squash and apple. If you don't have an immersion blender, then just remove the squash and apple pieces and puree in a blender or food processor and then pour back into the pot.

6. Mix in the cinnamon, nutmeg, cloves, and salt to taste.

7. Enjoy!!

CHAPTER 4

Entree Recipes

This chapter has 10 amazing reecipes for you to enjoy

.

1. Slow Cooker Pal Beef Stew

Output: 4-6 bowls

Servings: 4

Estimated Time for preparation: 8 hours 20 minutes

Ingredients:

- 2 white parsnips, chopped
- 2 sweet potatoes, chopped
- 1 small onion, chopped
- 4 celery sticks, chopped
- 2 cloves of garlic, minced
- 2 lbs beef, cubed
- 4 carrots, chopped
- 1 14.5oz can of broth (beef, chicken, or vegetable or use water)
- 2 teaspoons of salt
- 1/2 teaspoon of black pepper

Directions:

1. Place everything into slow cooker, mix together, and cook for 8 hours on low temperature setting.

2. Serve your meal and enjoy

2. Slow Cooker Bacon and Chicken

Output: 4 plates

Servings: 4

Estimated Time for preparation: 8 hours 5 minutes

Ingredients:

- 10 slices of bacon (uncooked), chopped into small pieces
- 5 chicken breasts
- 2 tablespoons thyme
- 1 tablespoon oregano
- 1 tablespoon rosemary (dried) (or use Italian seasoning instead of separate herbs)
- 5 tablespoons olive oil

Directions:

1. Place everything into slow cooker, mix together, and cook for 8 hours on the low temperature setting. Add only 2 tablespoons of olive oil first.

2. Shred the meat and mix with 3 tablespoons of olive oil.

3. Enjoy your soup

3. Pineapple Pork with Garlic and Cilantro

Output: 2 bowls

Servings: 2

Estimated Time of preparation: 15 minutes

Ingredients:

- 1 teaspoon freshly grated ginger
- 3 cloves of garlic, minced
- 2 cups of pineapple chunks (frozen or fresh)
- 3 cups of cooked shredded pork (or chicken) (pork or chicken made in advance in a slow cooker)
- 1/4 cup of cilantro, chopped
- Salt and pepper to taste
- Coconut oil to cook in

Directions:

1. Melt 1 tablespoon of coconut oil in a saucepan and add in the pineapple chunks.

2. Drop in the shredded pork and heat for about 5 minutes.

3. Add in the ginger, garlic, cilantro, and season with salt and pepper to taste.

4. Enjoy

4. Pan-Fried Tilapia with Coconut Carrot Mash and Garlic Zucchini Sauté

Estimated Time for preparation: 30 minutes

Output: Two plates

Servings: 2

Ingredients:

- 2 tablespoons coconut milk
- 2 tilapia filets
- 2 tablespoons coconut oil for frying
- 2 cups carrots, peeled and shredded
- 1 zucchini, thinly sliced
- 3 cloves garlic, minced
- Salt to taste
- Olive oil for frying

Directions:

1. Dress the zucchini with the garlic and olive oil. Salt to taste.

2. Boil the carrots in a pot of water until tender (drain and puree). Mix with the coconut milk.

3. Pan-fry the tilapia in coconut oil – let it cook until most of the fish has turned from opaque to white.

4. Use a flat spatula to flip the filets over carefully and let it cook for a few more minutes.

5. Add salt to taste.

6. Serve and enjoy

5. Pan-Fried Pork Tenderloin with Peach and Basil Sauce

Estimated time for preparation: 30 minutes

Yield: 2 plates

Servings: 2

Ingredients:

- 1 lb pork tenderloin
- 4 basil leaves
- 2 tablespoons coconut oil
- 1 teaspoon raw honey (optional)
- salt and pepper to taste
- 1 tablespoon coconut oil
- 2 peaches, peel and chop into pieces

Directions:

1. Cut the 1 lb pork tenderloin in half.

2. Put the 1 tablespoon of coconut oil measured into a frying pan on a medium heat and fry the two pork tenderloin pieces in the pan.

3. Be sure to attend to the frying pan so as the pork won't get burnt. As one side cooks, use a tong to flip the other side to cook. Repeat till it's throughly done.

4. Cook all sides of the pork until the meat thermometer shows an internal temperature of just below 145F (63C). The pork will keep on cooking a bit after you take it out of the pan.

5. While the pork is cooking, puree the peach pieces, basil leaves, 2 tablespoons of coconut oil, and the raw honey.

6. Let the pork sit for a few minutes and then slice into 1-inch thick slices with a sharp knife.

7. Serve with the peach and basil sauce.

8. Enjoy

5. Grilled Chicken Drumsticks with Garlic Marinade

Estimated time for preparation: 30 minutes

Output: Ten drumsticks

Servings: 2

Ingredients:

- 1/2 cups of olive oil
- 1 head of garlic (around 10 cloves)
- juice from 1 lemon
- 10 chicken drumsticks
- 1 tablespoon of sea salt
- 1/2 teaspoon of pepper

Directions:

1. Put the lemon juice, sea salt, olive oil, garlic, and pepper into a blender or food processor and puree. This is the marinade.

2. Rub the chicken drumsticks in the marinade.

3. Grill the chicken drumsticks and make sure it cooks well.

4. Enjoy.

6. Saffron Orange Acorn Squash Mash with Bacon and Collard Greens

Estimated Time of preparation: 1 hour

Output: 4 bowls

Servings: 4

Ingredients:

- 10 oz collard greens (approx. 1 bunch)
- 2 medium-sized acorn squash (or 1 butternut squash)
- 1/2 navel orange, finely chopped
- 1 lb bacon, diced
- Pinch of saffron (crush and soak for 30 minutes in warm water)

Directions:

1. Preheat the oven to 400F.

2. Divide the acorn squash into two and remove the seeds.

3. Bake the squash on a baking tray in the oven for 40 minutes at 400F (200C) or microwave on high for 3 minutes to soften the inside of the squash

4. Cook the bacon in a pot until fine.

5. Boil the collard greens in a pot of boiling water for 40 minutes until tender.

5. Scoop out the inside of the acorn squash when it's tender. Place the soft scooped-out acorn squash flesh into the pot with the beef bacon and the collard greens.

6. Add the orange and saffron (optional) to the pot and cook on a low heat for about 5-10 minutes until the acorn squash forms a fine mash.

7. Divide the "mash" into four bowls to serve.

8. Enjoy

7. Braised Cardamom Cabbage and Pork

Estimated Time for preparation: 2 hours 15 minutes

Yield: 4 bowls

Servings: 4

Ingredients:

- 1 lb pork (tenderloin or other cut), diced
- 1/2 tablespoon cardamom powder
- 1 teaspoon turmeric
- 1 head of cabbage, sliced
- 1 leek, sliced (or use an onion)
- 1 apple, peeled, cored, and diced
- 1 cup (16oz or 500ml) chicken broth (or 500 ml water)
- salt to taste
- coconut oil to cook with

Directions:

1. Put two tablespoons of coconut oil into a large saucepan on high heat.

2. Wait till the oil is heat up, then add in the diced pork and sear the pork.

3. When all the pork pieces are cooked and browned, add in the chicken stock, cabbage, leek, apple, and spices.

4. Cover the saucepan and allow to cook for about 1 hour 30 minutes. Stir occasionally to ensure nothing sticks to the bottom of the saucepan.

5. The food is done when the pork is soft and tender. Add salt to taste.

6. Serve and enjoy

8. Thai Chicken and Cauliflower Rice

Estimated Time for preparation: 30 minutes

Output: four bowls

Servings: 4

Ingredients:

- 3 cloves of garlic, crushed
- meat from a whole chicken, shredded (you can use the chicken meat from the Slow Cooker Thai Chicken Soup)
- 1 head of cauliflower
- 1 tablespoon freshly grated ginger
- coconut oil to cook with
- 1 tablespoon coconut aminos (optional)
- 1/2 cup cilantro, chopped (for garnish)
- Salt

Directions:

1. Break the cauliflower into florets and process until it forms a rice-like texture. This may be done in bit by bit to achieve desired result.

2. Put coconut oil into a large pan

3. Put the cauliflower into a large pan with coconut oil and cook the cauliflower rice (may need to be done in 2 pans or in batches). Keep the heat on medium and stir regularly.

3. Add in the measured ginger and garlic.

4. Observe the food, when the cauliflower rice is soft, add in the shredded chicken meat.

5. Add in the coconut aminos and salt to taste. Mix well.

6. Top with cilantro.

7. Best served with a bowl of slow cooker Thai chicken soup.

8. Enjoy

9. Cauliflower Crusted Pizza topped with Spinach and Prosciutto

Estimated Time for preparation: 35 minutes

Output: 6 pizzas

Servings: 2

Ingredients:

- 4 handfuls of spinach leaves
- 1/2 head cauliflower
- 8 tablespoons olive oil
- 1 tablespoon garlic powder
- 1 tablespoon Italian seasoning
- 1/2 teaspoon salt
- 12 slices of prosciutto or ham (make sure there are no AIP-forbidden ingredients in the meat – check when you purchase it or alternatively top with chicken or othermeat)
- olive oil for greasing

Directions:

1. Break the cauliflower into pieces, and process the cauliflower with the 8 tablespoons olive oil, garlic powder, Italian season, and salt until it forms a soft mash

2. Preheat oven to 350F. Line a baking tray with parchment paper and then grease it with some olive oil.

3. Squeeze the water out of the cauliflower mash.

4. Then divide the mash into six parches.

5. Cup each mash into a small pizza dough and bake in the oven for 20 minutes until the crust turns slightly brown and harder.

6. While the crust is baking, boil a pot of water and drop the spinach into the boiling water. Boil for about a minute and remove the spinach.

7. Place 2 slices of prosciutto onto each pizza (to prevent the spinach from making it soggy) then place the spinach on top.

8. Eat off the parchment paper as the crust is too fragile to remove.

9. Enjoy

10. Baked Salmon on a bed of Cabbage, Fennel, and Apple

Estimated Time for preparation: 40 minutes

Output: 4 plates

Servings: 4

Ingredients:

- 1/2 cup chicken broth (or water)
- 4 tablespoons of coconut oil
- 3-4 slices of bacon, chopped into pieces (optional)
- 4 salmon filets
- 8 tablespoons olive oil
- 1/2 head of cabbage, chopped into small pieces
- 1 head of fennel, diced (or use 1 celery heart)
- 2 apples, peeled and diced
- Pepper
- Salt

Directions:

1. Preheat oven to 350F.

2. Place each salmon filet onto a piece of aluminum foil with 2 tablespoons of olive oil and sprinkle with a bit of salt and pepper.

3. Wrap up the aluminum foils and place in the oven for 30 minutes.

4. Put the coconut oil into a large saucepan and add in the cabbage and chicken broth and put the lid on the saucepan, allow to cook for about 10 minutes.

5. Put in the fennel, stir and cover the saucepan, cook for another 10 minutes.

6. Put in the apples. Stir and season with salt and pepper to taste. Cook until the salmon is done.

7. Place the cabbage mixture on a plate, place the salmon on top, then top with bacon pieces.

8. Enjoy

CHAPTER 4

Side Dish Recipes

This chapter has 7 amazing simple and fast recipes for you to enjoy.

1. Ginger and Garlic Bok Choy Sauté

Estimated Time for preparation: 15 minutes

Output: 1 plate

Servings: 2

Ingredients:

- 5 bunches of Bok Chok
- 2 cloves of garlic, minced
- 1 teaspoon fresh ginger, grated
- salt
- coconut oil for cooking

Directions:

1. Cut off the ends of the bok choy.

2. Then chop the bok choy into 1-inch long chunks.

3. Put 1 tablespoon of coconut oil into a saucepan on a medium heat.

4. Put in the bok choy chunks into the saucepan. Stir frequently while the bok choy cooks.

5. After the bok choy starts to wilt, mix in the garlic, ginger, and salt to taste.

6. Leave to cook for about 1-2 minutes more and serve.

7. Enjoy

2. Endives and Pear Sauté

Estimated Time for preparation: 15 minutes

Output: 1 plate

Servings: 2

Ingredients:

- 2 cloves garlic, minced
- 1 teaspoon apple cider vinegar
- 4 endives, chopped into 1-inch chunks
- 1 pear, peeled and diced
- Coconut oil for cooking
- Salt for seasoning

Directions:

1. Place 1 tablespoon of coconut oil into a frying pan on medium heat and add the endives.

2. As soon as the endives start wilting a bit, add the minced garlic, diced pear, vinegar, and salt. Make sure to mix well.

3. Cook for 2 minutes and serve.

3. Roasted Turmeric Cauliflower

Estimated Time for preparation: 150 minutes

Output: 1 large bowl

Servings: 4

Ingredients:

- Half of a large head of cauliflower
- 2 teaspoons of turmeric
- 2 teaspoons of salt
- 2 tablespoons of olive oil

Directions:

1. Preheat oven to 350F (175C).

2. Pull off florets from the cauliflower and mix with the turmeric, salt, and olive oil.

3. Put the mixture in baking dish, make sure to spread the cauliflower so they don't lap on top of each other.

4. Cover the baking dish with tin foil, and bake for about an 1 hour 20 minutes.

5. Enjoy

4. Easy Bacon Brussels Sprouts

Estimated Time for preparation: 25 minutes

Output: 1 very large bowl

Servings: 4-6

Ingredients:

- 2 lbs Brussels sprouts
- 1 lb bacon, uncooked (chopped into small pieces)

Directions:

1. Chop off the ends from the Brussels sprouts and chop each in half.

2. Boil the halved Brussels sprouts for 10 minutes until tender.

3. While the Brussels sprouts are boiling, chop the bacon into small pieces (approx. 1/2-inch wide), and cook the bacon pieces in a separate large pot on medium heat. When the bacon is crispy, add in the drained Brussels sprouts (so that the Brussels sprouts are in the pot with the bacon fat).

4. Cook for 10 more minutes, mixing occasionally to make sure nothing gets burnt on the bottom of the pan.

5. Enjoy

5. Lemon Asparagus Sauté with Bacon Topping

Estimated Time for preparation: 20 minutes

Output : 1 large bowl

Servings: 2-4

Yield: 1 large bowl

Servings: 2-4

Total Time: 20 minutes

Ingredients:

- 20 stalks of asparagus (approx.), chop off the end of the stalks and chop into small chunks
- 1 lemon
- 1/2 cup bacon bits/pieces, precooked
- salt to taste
- Olive oil or bacon fat to cook with

Directions:

1. Sauté the asparagus in 2 tablespoons of olive oil.

2. When the asparagus slices are tender, squeeze in the juice from 1 lemon. Add just about how much lemon juice you like.

3. Add in the bacon bits and sauté for 2-3 minutes more.

4. Add salt to taste.

5. Enjoy

6. Baked Parsnip Fries with Parsley

Estimated Time for preparation: 50 minutes

Output: 1 large bowl

Servings: 4

Ingredients:

- 4 parsnips, peeled and cut into fries
- 1/4 cup parsley, finely chopped
- 1/4 cup olive oil
- 1 tablespoon salt
- 1 teaspoon black pepper

Directions:

1. Preheat oven to 450F.

2. Toss all the ingredients together in a large bowl and spread the fries onto a baking tray.

3. Bake for 40 minutes. Make sure to stir the fries around after 20 minutes to ensure they don't burn.

4. Enjoy

7. Coconut Mashed Sweet Potatoes with Shredded Coconut and Ginger

Estimated Time for preparation: 35 minutes/1 hour 10 minutes depending on method of cooking

Output: large bowl

Servings: 4

Ingredients:

- 1 cup coconut milk
- 4 sweet potatoes
- 1 teaspoon of ginger
- 2 tablespoons shredded coconut to dress.

Directions:

1. Bake the sweet potatoes for about 1 hour at 350F or boil or steam the sweet potatoes for about 30 mins. Make sure they are very tender - you will know they are tender when you are able to poke a fork into them with ease.

2. Let the sweet potatoes cool for a bit and then peel them.

3. Put the peeled sweet potatoes into a food processor with the coconut milk and ginger, and food process on high until smooth.

4. Enjoy

CHAPTER 5

Snack Recipes

This chapter has 7 amazing simple and fast recipes for you to enjoy.

1. Baked Sweet Potato Chips

Estimated Time for preparation: 40 minutes

Output: 1 large bowl

Servings: 4

Ingredients:

- 2 large sweet potatoes, finely sliced
- 1 tablespoon coconut oil
- 1 teaspoon salt

Directions:

1. Preheat oven to 400F.

2. Sprinkle the coconut oil and salt on the sweet potatoes.

3. Spread in a single layer on 2 baking trays.

4. Bake them for about 35 minutes. Make sure to flip after about 15 minutes to avoid burning.

5. Enjoy

2. Avocado Bacon Cups

Estimated time for preparation: 45 minutes

Output: 12 cups

Servings: 12

Ingredients:

- 30 thin slices of bacon
- 2 ripe avocados
- Olive oil
- Balsamic vinegar
- Salt for seasoning
- For this you would need a standard nonstick metal muffin or cupcake pan

Directions:

1. Preheat oven to 400F.

2. Use 2 and 1/2 slices of bacon to make one bacon cup.

3. Turn the muffin cup over to the reverse side, and place 2 half slices of bacon across the back of one of the muffin cups. Place another half slice across those 2, just in between those first 2 half slices. Then wrap a whole slice around the cup tightly.

4. Repeat for the other cups.

5. Bake for about 25 minutes until crispy. Watch for any dripping fat underneath the oven and place a baking tray underneath in the oven to catch any dripping bacon fat.

6. Cool for 5-10 minutes and then carefully remove the bacon cups from the back of the muffin tray. Store in the fridge until you're ready to enjoy (up to a week).

7. Make the avocado filling when you're ready to eat.

8. To do this, cut the avocado into cubes and sprinkle with olive oil, balsamic vinegar, and salt to taste.

9. Place into the bacon cups.

10. Enjoy

3. Dehydrated Fruits and Vegetables

Dehydrated fruits and vegetables are very handy snacks, you can eat them as veggie or fruit chips. One of the best part of dehydrating your fruits and vegetables is much more longer shelf life of the dehydrated chips, which means you can dehydrate them, store and munch away whenever you want to.

For vegetables (e.g. pumpkin), slice them into thin slices so it's faster to dry. Salting them (or dipping the slices into salt water) also makes them dry faster.

For fruits, slice thin as well. Wash and peel if necessary. Dehydration times using a dehydrator vary (longer from fruits generally). Check after 8-10 hours.

Personal Suggestion: You might not want to dehydrate onions, they usually give out a strong smell which will cover the house. You can get dried onions in the spice section of food stores and they are cheap too.

4. Coconut Plantains Chips

Estimatedl Time for preparation: 45 minutes

Output: 1 bowl

Servings: 2

Ingredients:

- 2 plantains, peeled and sliced really thin
- coconut oil for frying
- salt for seasoning

Directions:

1. Put the coconut oil into a saucepan so that it's about one fourth of the pan.

2. Heat up the oil for 3-4 minutes on a medium heat.

3. Put in the plantain slices one by one into the oil so they're not overlapping ie touching each other. Put in as much slices the saucepan can contain at a time.

4. Use a perforated spoon to get the slices out as soon as they turn golden.

5. Repeat until all the slices are fried.

6. Toss the chips with salt to taste.

7. Enjoy your chips.

5. Salt and Vinegar Kale Chips

Estimated Time for preparation: 20 minutes or 5 hours, depending on the method of cooking.

Yield: 1 bowl

Servings: 1-2

Ingredients:

- 1 teaspoon apple cider vinegar
- 4 large kale leaves
- 1/2 tablespoon salt
- 2 tablespoons olive oil

Directions:

1. Wash the kale leaves and remove the stem so you're just left with leaves.

2. Dry the leaves well.

3. Get a big bowl and add the leaves with the olive oil, salt and vinegar and mix well with a spatula.

4. If using the dehydrator, place the kale leaves flat on the dehydrator trays (with no overlapping) and dehydrate until crispy on 135F (3-5 hours).

If using the oven, then preheat oven to 300F and place the leaves flat on a baking tray (with no overlapping). Bake for 5-10 minutes - make sure the leaves get crispy but not burned.

If using a microwave, place the kale leaves on a microwavable plate and place in microwave on full power for 2-3 minutes (check after 2 minutes to make sure they aren't burning).

5. Enjoy your chips

CHAPTER 6

Dessert

This chapter has 7 amazing simple and fast recipes for you to enjoy.

1. Raw Carrot Cake

Estimated Time for preparation: 2 hours 10 minutes

Output: 12 pieces

Servings: 4

Ingredients:

- 1/4 cup raw honey
- 1 tablespoon coconut oil
- 1 teaspoon vanilla extract
- 1 teaspoon lemon juice
- 1 teaspoon cinnamon
- 1 cup carrots, finely chopped
- 1/2 cup shredded coconut
- 1 teaspoon freshly grated ginge
- 1/2 teaspoon nutmeg
- Dash of cloves

Directions:

1. Press all the ingredients into a baking dish or just form using your hand into uniform 1-inch thick layer.

2. Refrigerate for 2-3 hours. Cut into squares or slices.

3. Enjoy

2. Apple Ginger Spice Sweet Potato Cookies

Estimated Time for preparation: 30 minutes

Output: 10-15 cookies

Servings: 4

Ingredients:

- 1 apple, peeled
- 1/2 cup shredded coconut
- 1 teaspoon freshly grated ginger
- 1 medium sweet potato, cooked and mashed
- 2 tablespoons raw honey
- 1 teaspoon cinnamon

Directions:

1. Preheat oven to 350F

2. Line a baking tray with parchment paper.

3. Using a blender, blend all the ingredients together.

4. Form small 2-inch diameter cookies, make them even but thin

5. Bake for 20-25 minutes, they are done when they are crisp and solid.

6. Enjoy

3. Cinnamon Pear and Butternut Squash Bowls

Estimated Time for preparation: 40 minutes

Output: 4 bowls

Servings: 4

Ingredients:

- 1 tablespoon cinnamon
- 1 butternut squash, diced into cubes
- 2 pears, peeled and dicced cubes
- 1 tablespoon raw honey
- Coconut oil for cooking
- Coconut cream to serve with (optional)

Directions:

1. Add 2-3 tablespoons of coconut oil in a large saucepan

2. Cook the butternut squash on for 10 minutes, stirring every few minutes. Make sure to cover the lid of the saucepan.

3. Add in the pears, raw honey, and cinnamon.

4. Cook until the pears and the butternut squash are tender.

5. Divide into bowls and serve with coconut cream.

6. Enjoy

4. 5-Minute Pumpkin Pie

Estimated Time for preparation: 5 minutes

Yield: 1 ramekin

Serves: 1

Ingredients:

- 1 teaspoon raw honey
- 6 tablespoons pumpkin puree
- 3 tablespoons coconut oil
- dash of cinnamon
- dash of nutmeg
- dash of cloves

Directions:

1. Put all the ingredients into a microwaveable bowl and microwave on high for 45 seconds. This will make it easier to blend.

2. Using a blender, blend well.

3. Serve immediately as it is or chill in refrigerator for it to be a bit solid.

4. Enjoy

5. Microwave Banana Bread

Estimated Time for preparation: 10 minutes

Output: 1 banana bread

Servings: 1

Ingredients:

- 2 1/2 tablespoons coconut oil, melted
- 1/2 teaspoon baking powder
- 1/4 cup coconut flour
- 1 ripe banana
- 1/2 teaspoon vanilla extract (optional)

Directions:

1. Mash the banana in a microwaveable cup with a fork.

2. Pour the other ingredients together into the microwaveable mug.

3. Microwave on high for about 2 minutes.

4. Let the bread cool for a few minutes. You can eat from the mug.

6. **Strawberry Banana Macaroons**

Estimated Time for preparation: 1 hour 10 minutes

Yield: 12 macaroons

Servings: 4

Ingredients:

- 1 cup shredded coconut
- 1 teaspoon vanilla extract
- 2 tablespoons raw honey
- 2 fresh strawberries, cut into 12 pieces
- 1 ripe banana
- 2 tablespoons coconut oil

Directions:

1. Mash together all the ingredients except strawberries - ie the banana, coconut, vanilla, honey, and coconut oil- .

2. Form into 12 balls.

3. Top each macaroon with a piece of strawberry.

4. Chill in the refrigerator for about 1 hour.

5. Enjoy

7. Vanilla Coconut Blueberry Bars

Estimated Time for preparation: 1 hour 10 minutes

Yield: 8 bars

Servings: 4

Ingredients:

- 1/2 cup fresh blueberries
- 1 cup coconut butter
- 2 tablespoons coconut oil
- 2 tablespoons raw honey
- 1 teaspoon vanilla extract
- 1/4 cup raisins (optional)

Directions:

1. Mildly melt the coconut butter, coconut oil, and honey to form a consistent mixture.

2. Add the vanilla extract into the mixture.

3. Line a baking tray with parchment paper and pour the mixture in.

4. Push the blueberries and raisins in and spread equally.

5. Chill in the refrigerator for about 1 hour.

6. Cut into bars.

7. Enjoy your dessert!!

8. Berry Jello

Estimated Time for preparation: 4 hours

Output: 2 cups

Servings: 2

Ingredients:

- 2 tablespoons of gelatin powder
- 1 cup of water
- 1 cup of strawberries
- 1 cup of blueberries
- 1 teaspoon raw honey (optional)

Directions:

1. Put the 2 tablespoons of the gelatin powder into a large bowl and add in 1 cup of cold water. Use a fork to stir very well to form a consistency.

2. Then place the bowl into the microwave and heat on high for 1 minute. Make sure to stir well to mix

3. Blend the strawberries and blueberries in a blender.

4. Pour the blended fruit into cups, upto half of the cup.

5. Pour the gelatin water into the cups with the fruit puree and fill up the cups.

5. Chill in the fridge to set for 3-4 hours.

6. Dress with a few slices of strawberries as toppings and serve.

7. Enjoy

9. Coconut Butter Stuffed Dates

Estimated Time for preparation: 10 minutes

Yield: 12 dates

Servings: 4

Ingredients:

- 1 cup coconut butter
- 12 pitted dates

Directions:

1. Slice open each date so that it opens out but isn't sliced in half.

2. Melt the coconut butter slightly in the microwave if it's not soft enough to scoop out with a spoon.

3. Stuff each date with as much coconut butter as you can fit in and as much as the space can contain.

4. Enjoy

10. Pineapple Mango Banana Sorbet

Estimated Time of preparation: 5 minutes

Output: 2 ramekins

Servings: 2

Ingredients:

- 1/2 tablespoon fresh lime juice
- 1/2 cup frozen pineapples
- 1 cup frozen mango pieces
- 1 banana, room temperature
- 1 banana for topping (optional)

Directions:

1. Put all the ingredients except the banana into a blender and blend really well. If your blender isnt that much strong, you can blend for a while and push the frozen fruits down to the bottom and continue blending. Make sure to blend well.

2. Top with a few banana slices.

3. Serve immediately.

4. Enjoy

ENJOY!!!